HEMATOLOGY & ONCOLOGY

for kids

Medical School
FOR KIDS™

First paperback edition June 2023

Book design by Betty Nguyen & Brandon Pham

ISBN 978-1-957557-15-1 (paperback)

Printed in the United States of America

Published by Black Phoenix Press

www.mdforkids.org

Disclaimer: Contents of this book are for informational purposes only. No material in this book is intended to provide, or be a substitute for, professional medical advice.

To the friends and family who have supported and loved us unconditionally, and to the mentors who have guided and taught us more than we could have imagined:

Thank you.

Betty & Brandon

Medical School
FOR KIDS™

Hematology & Oncology

(hee-muh-TAA-luh-jee & aang-KAA-luh-jee)

the branch of medicine concerned with the study and treatment of blood diseases, bleeding disorders, and cancer

Medical School FOR KIDS™

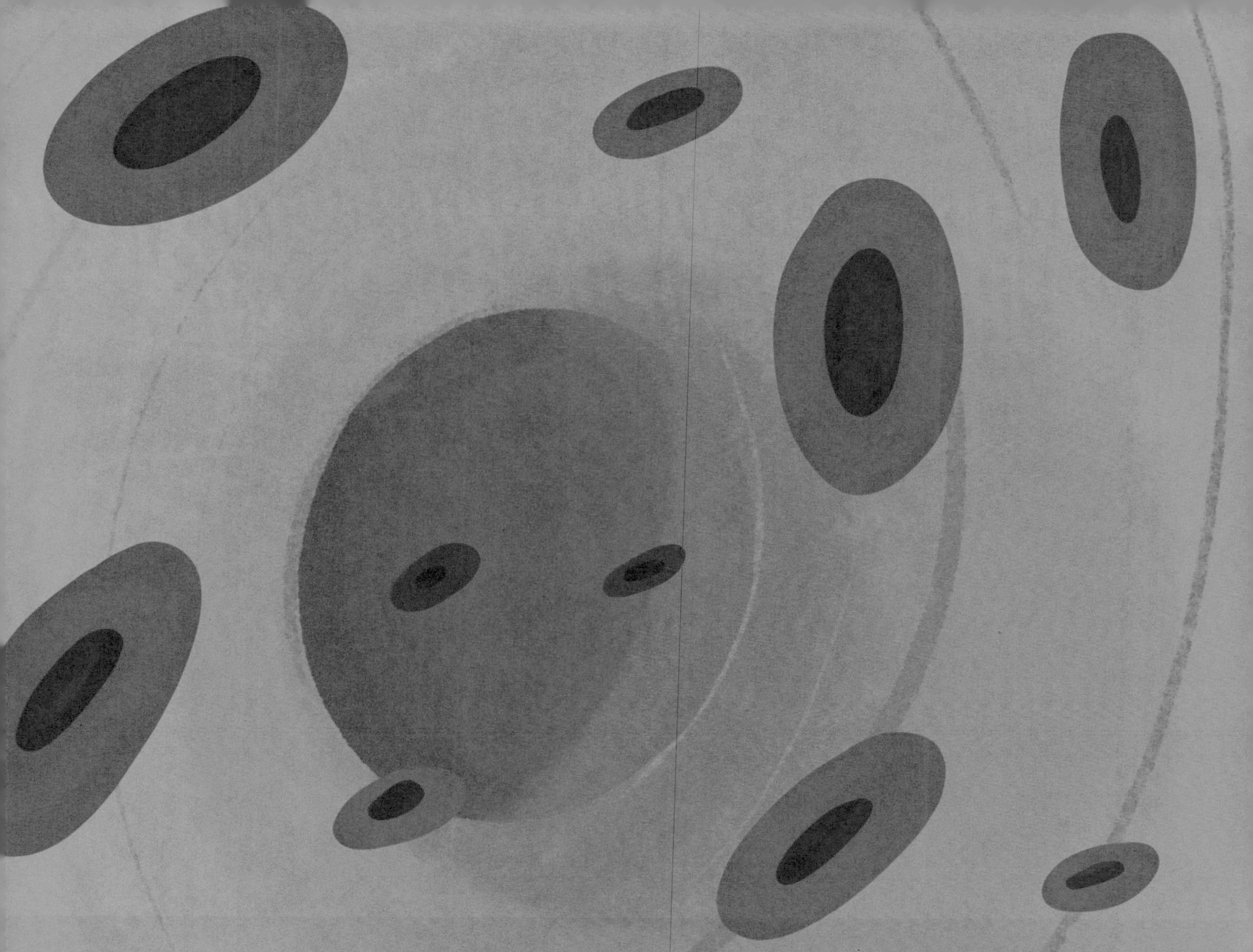

Blood is a red liquid that travels through our blood vessels and carries important substances to the rest of our bodies.

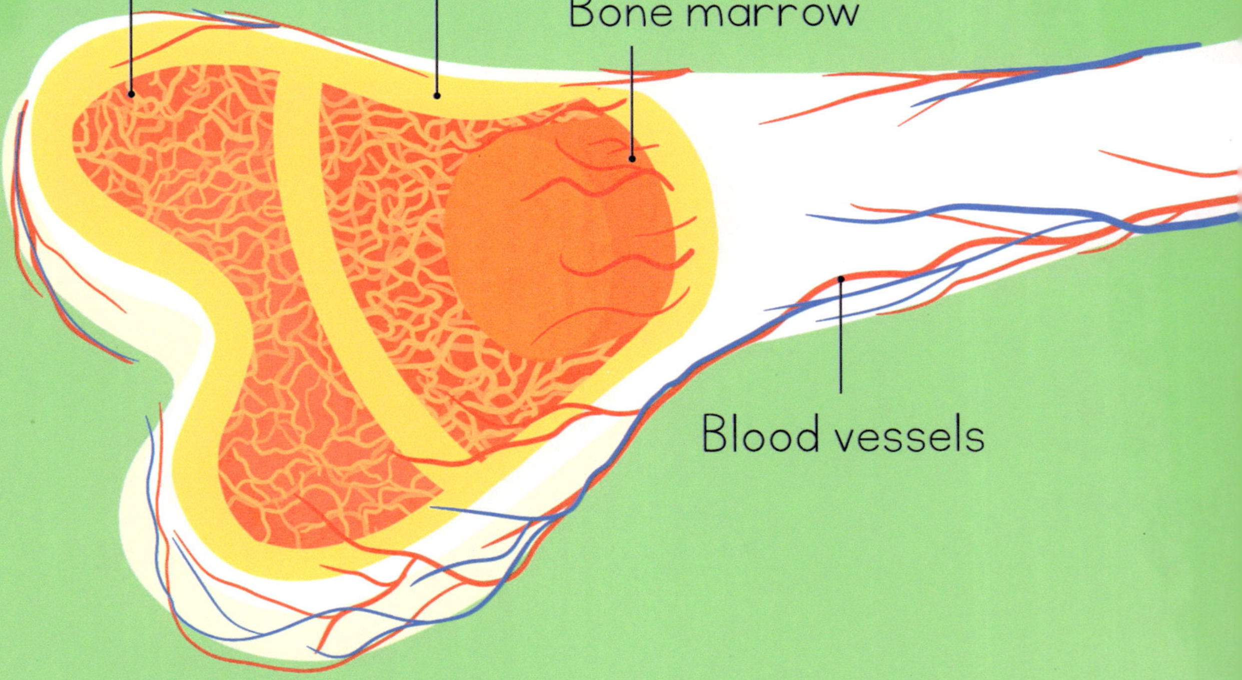

Cells in our blood develop from **hematopoietic stem cells**, which are made in a soft, spongy tissue inside our bones called **bone marrow**.

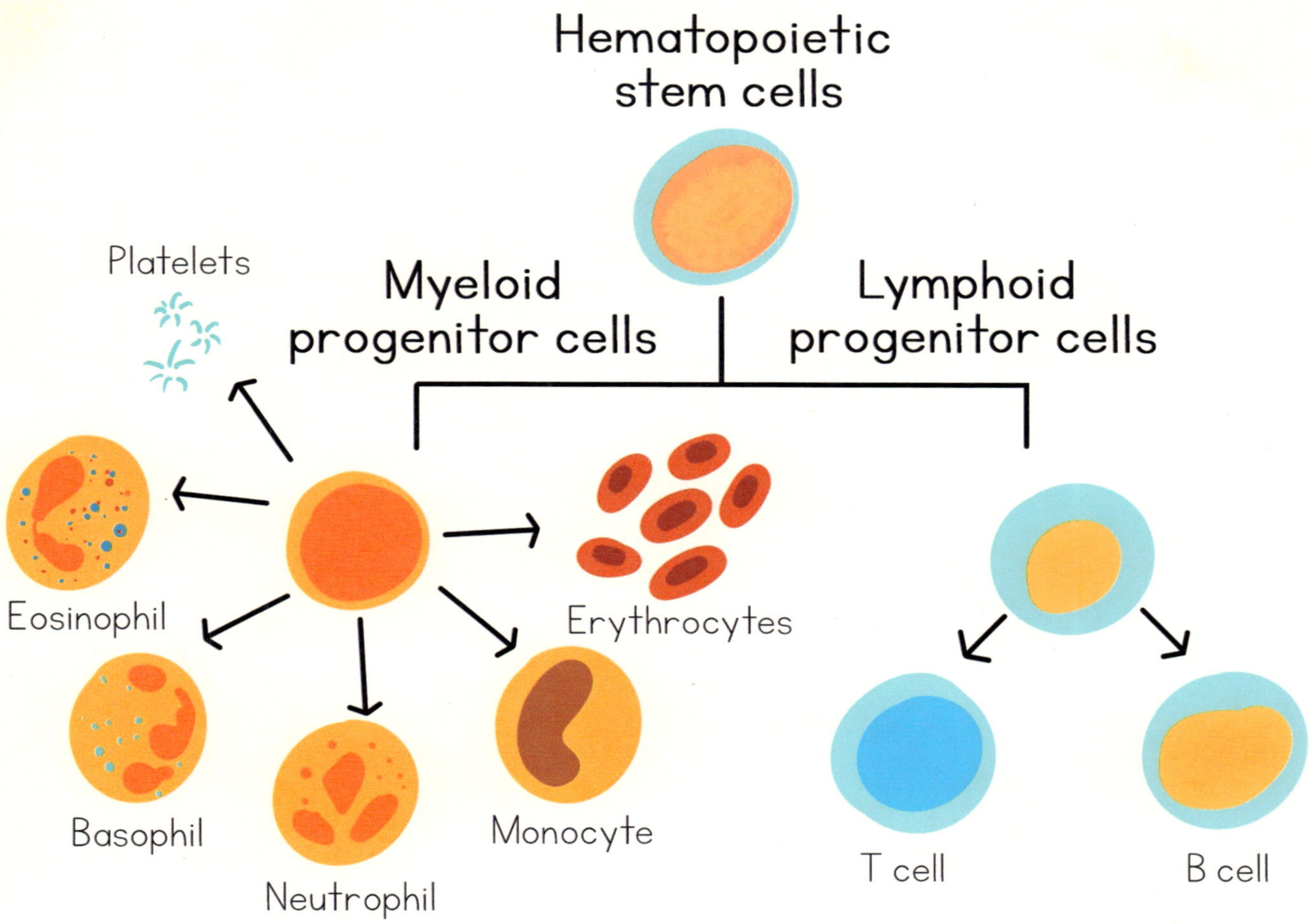

Hematopoietic stem cells develop into **myeloid** or **lymphoid progenitor cells**, which can then mature into many types of cells!

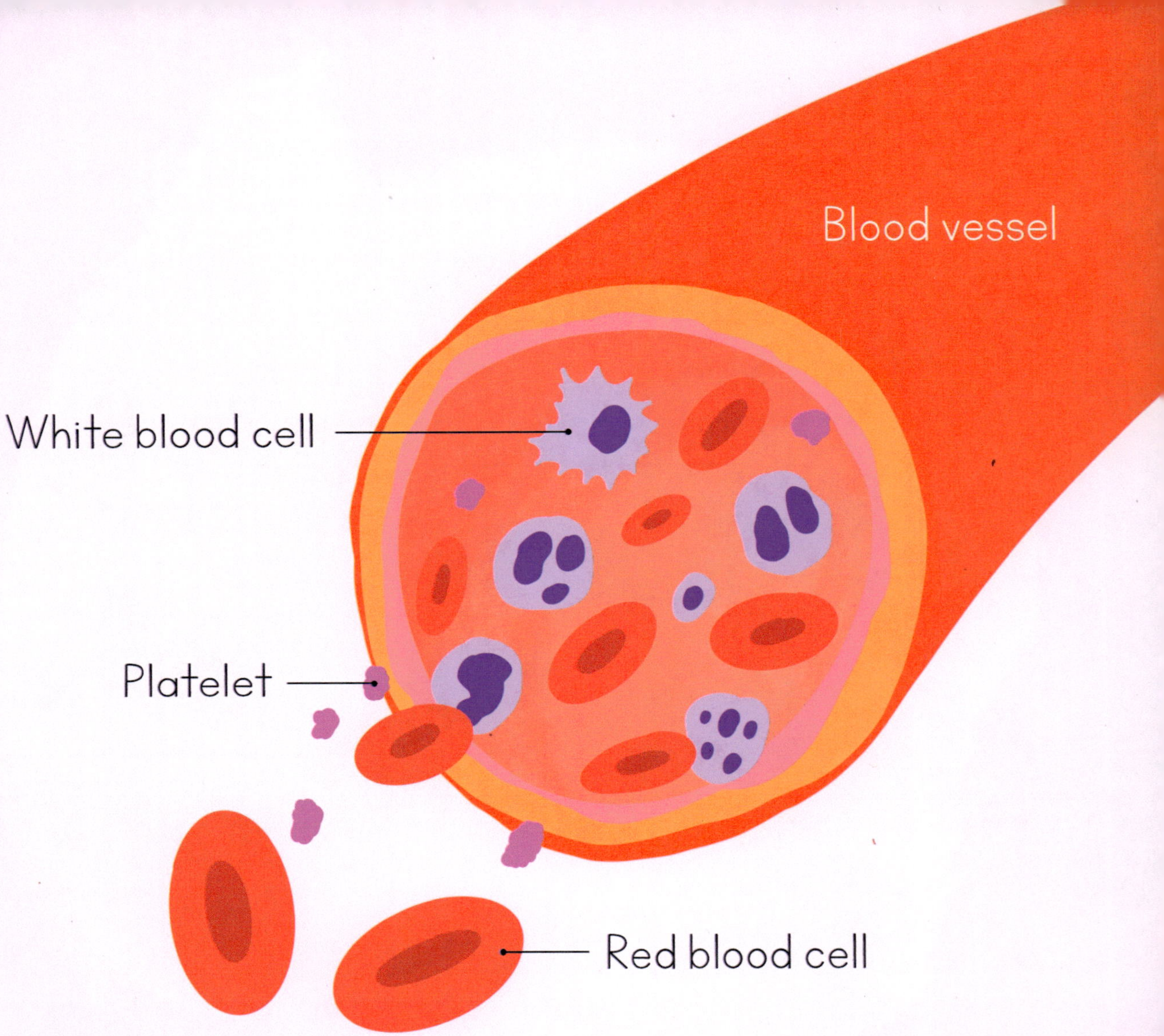

The three main types of cells in our blood are **red blood cells**, **platelets**, and **white blood cells**.

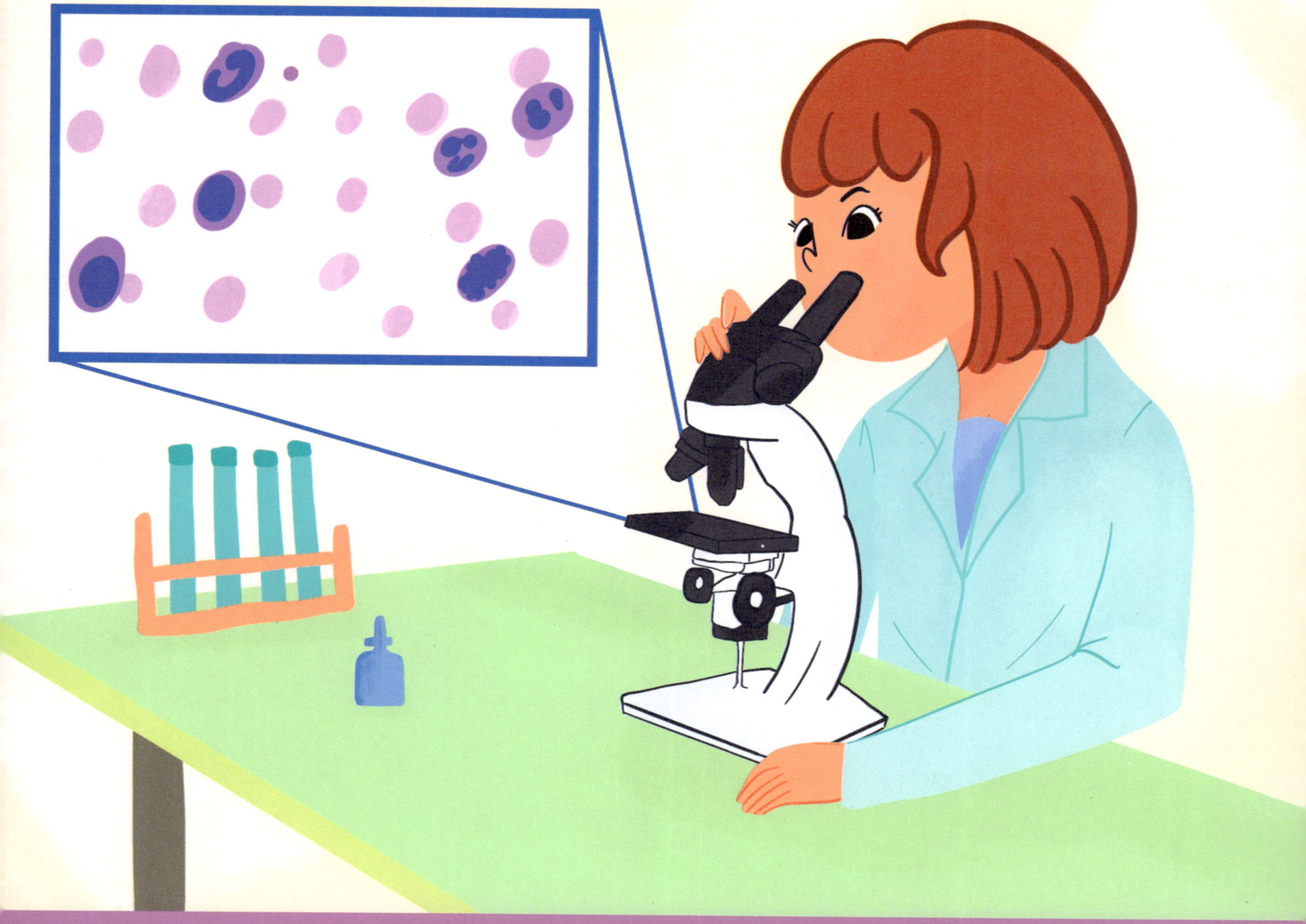

Doctors can look at these cells by smearing blood onto a glass slide and looking at it under a microscope. This is called a **blood smear**.

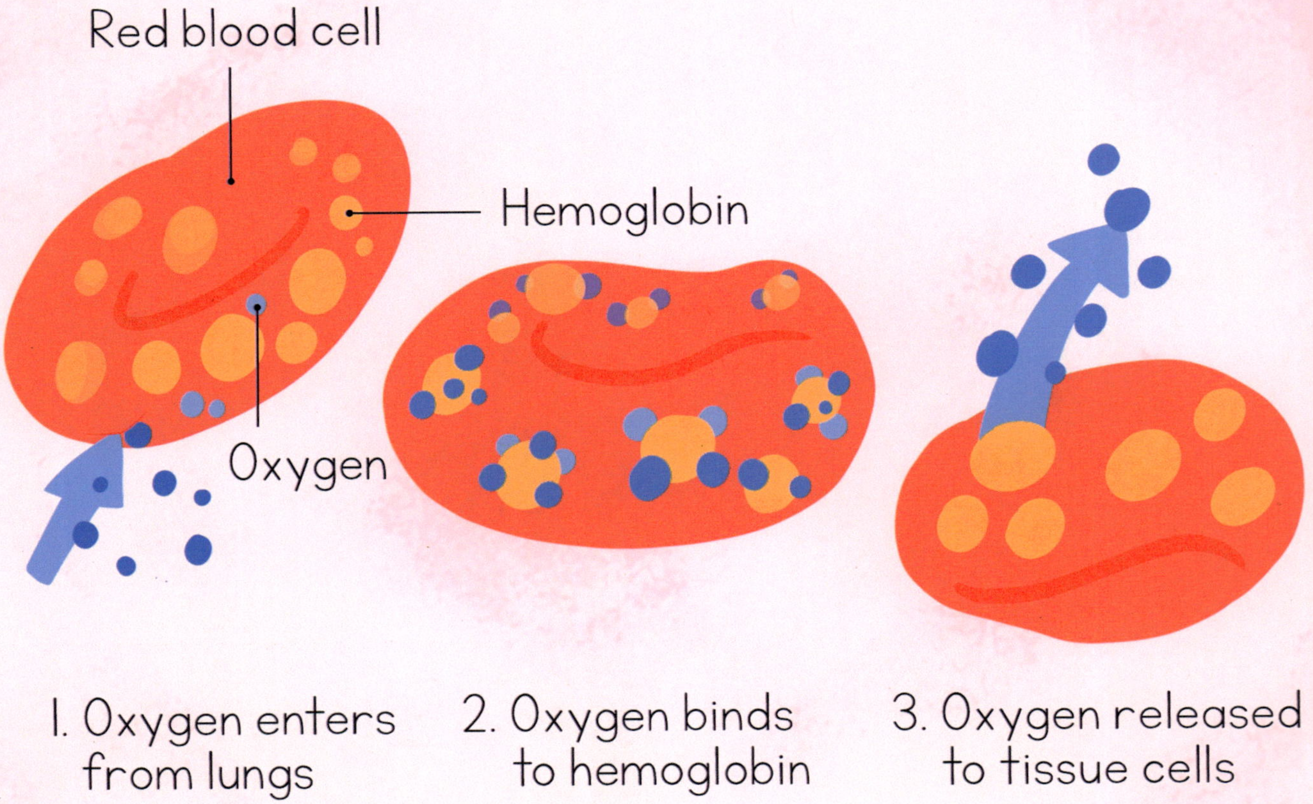

Red blood cells transport oxygen from our lungs to the rest of our body. **Hemoglobin** is a protein in red blood cells that binds to oxygen.

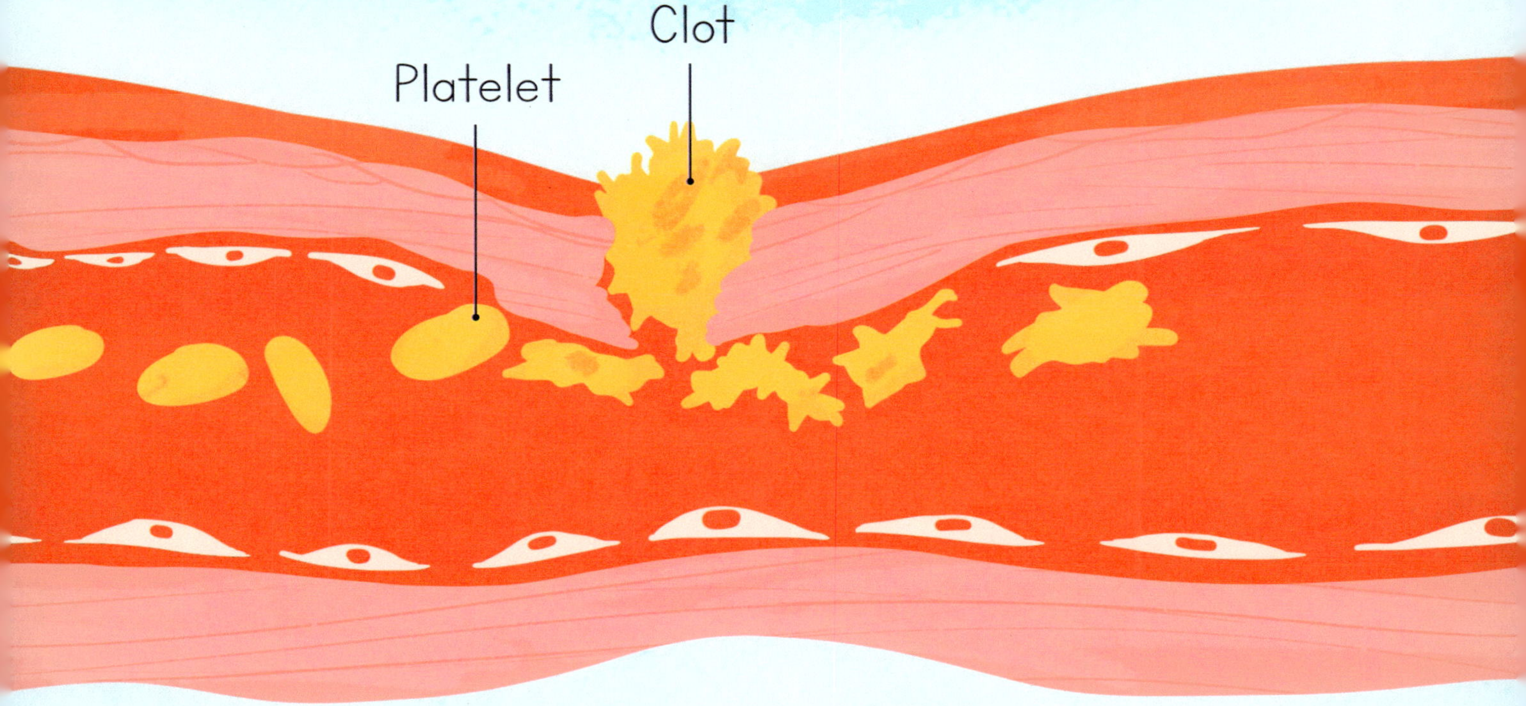

Platelets prevent and stop bleeding. Platelets do this by sticking to each other to form a clot.

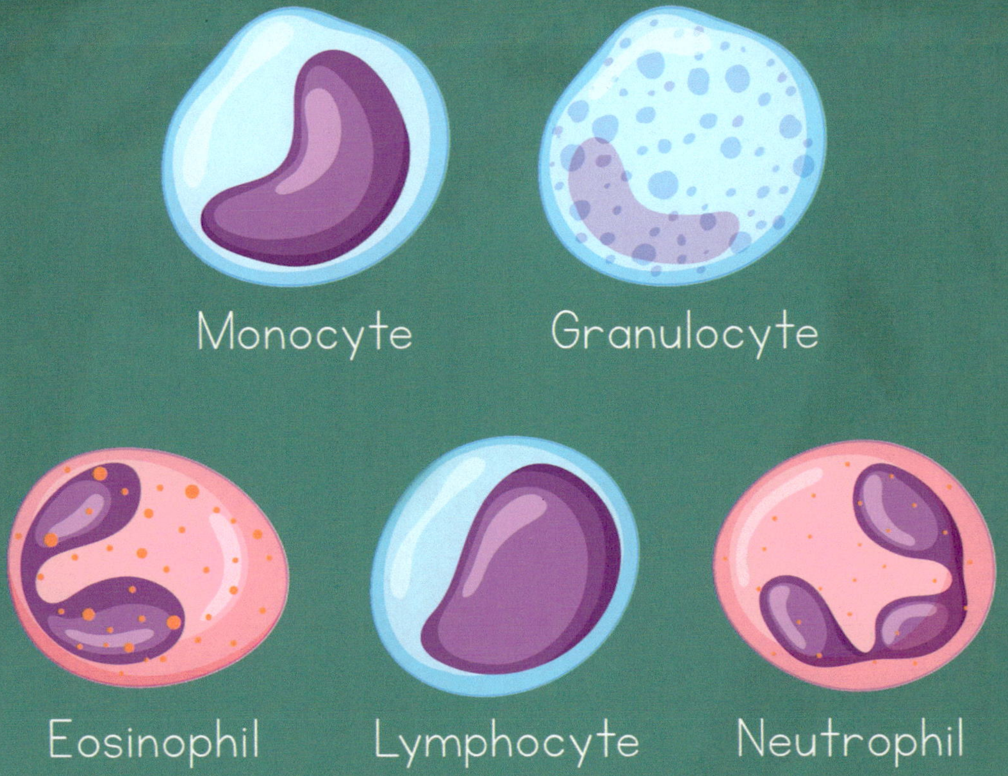

White blood cells help our body fight infections and other diseases. There are many types of white blood cells!

Complete blood count (CBC)

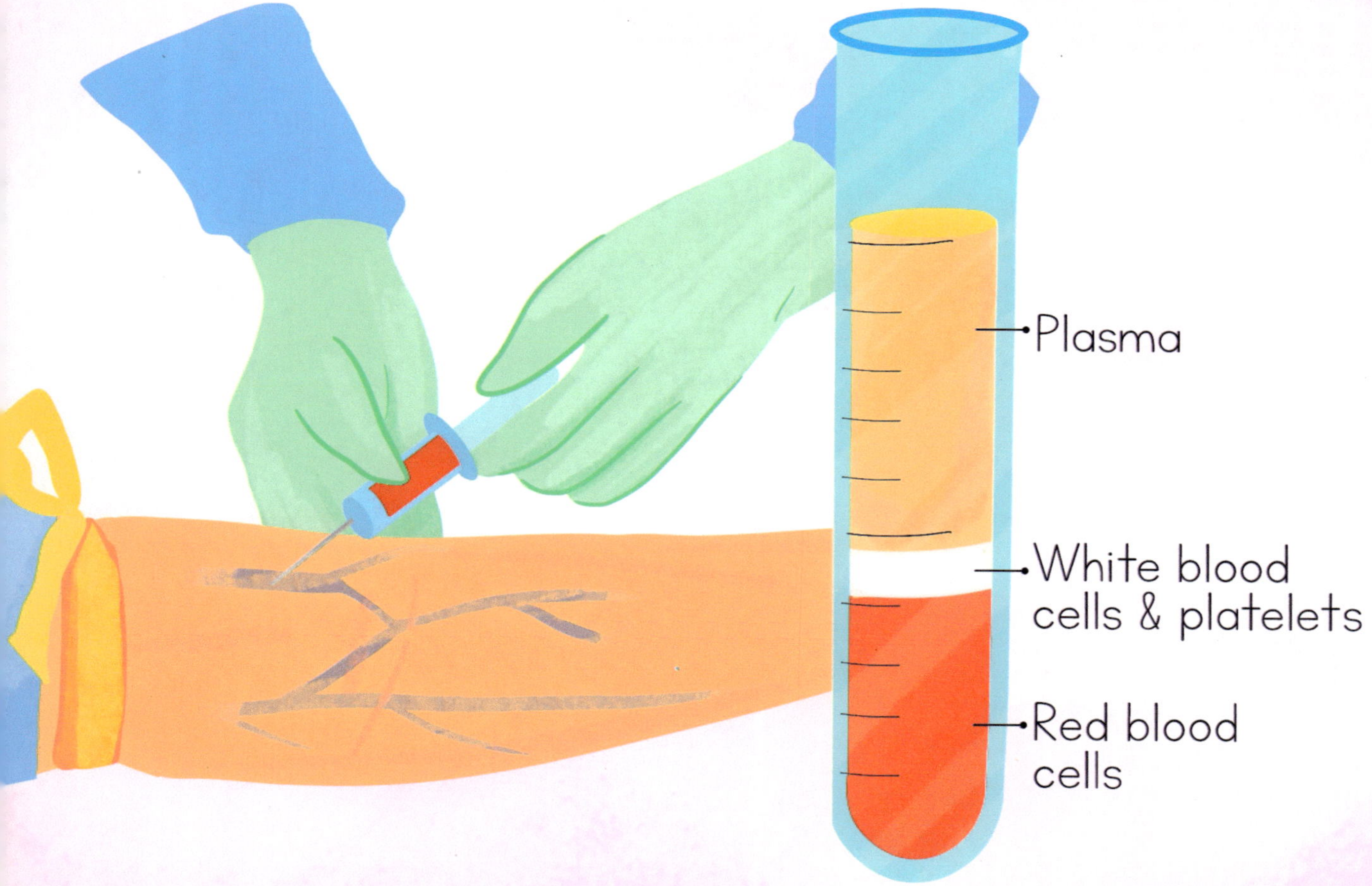

Doctors can measure the amounts of these cells in our blood using a blood test called a **complete blood count (CBC)**.

Symptoms of anemia

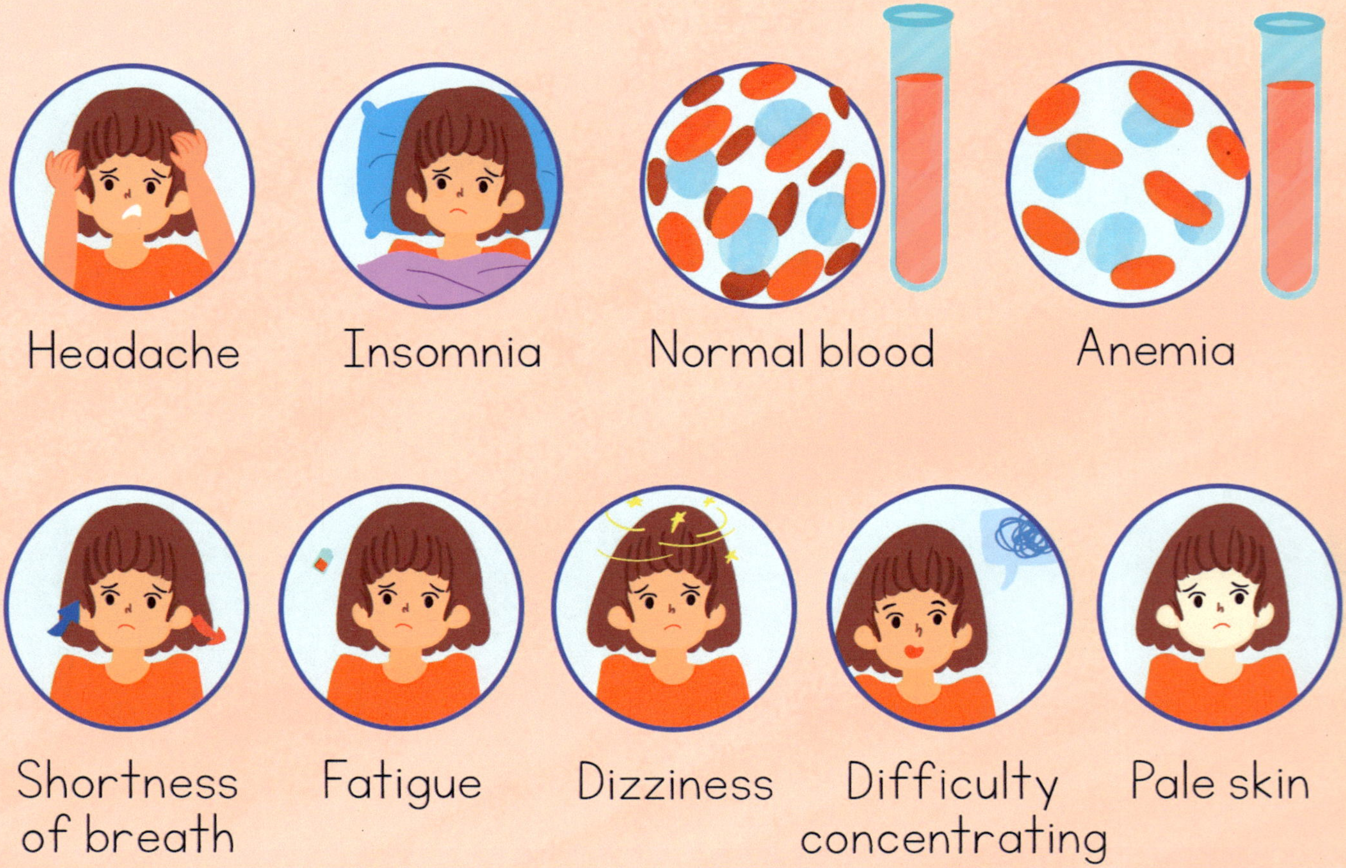

Having too few red blood cells is called **anemia.** This can cause patients to feel tired, weak, or dizzy.

Foods rich in iron, folate, and vitamin B12

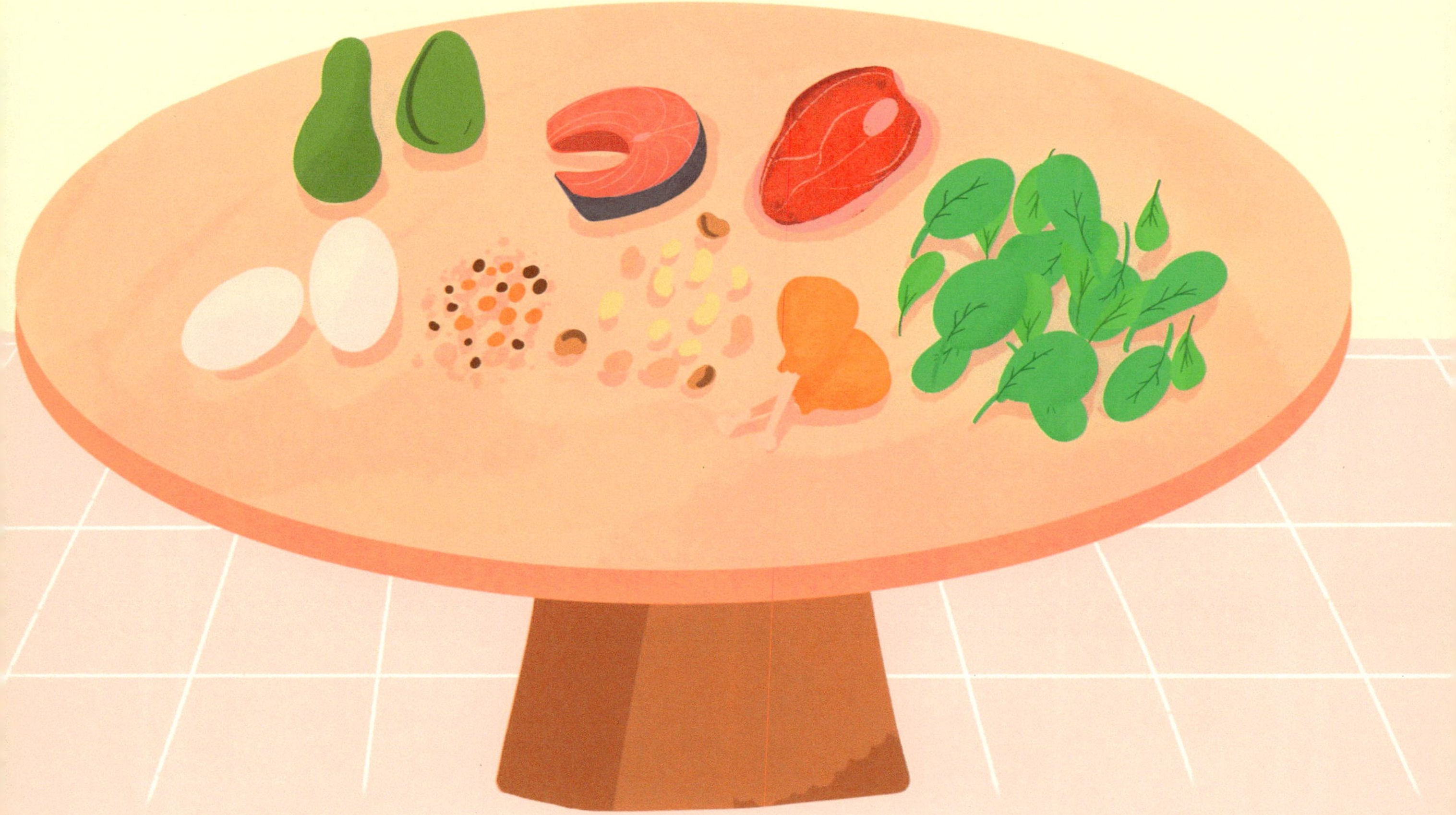

Some patients develop anemia because their body doesn't have enough nutrients, such as **iron**, **folate**, and **vitamin B12**, that are needed for red blood cells to grow.

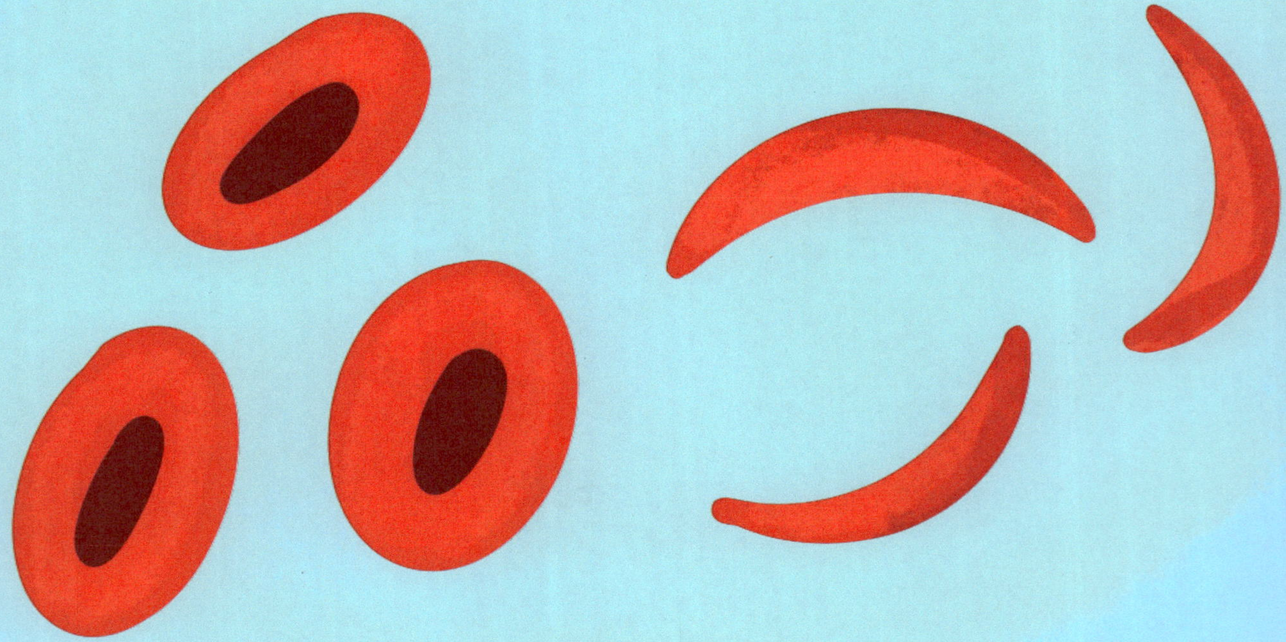

Other patients develop anemia because their red blood cells are crescent-shaped instead of round, causing them to break down faster. This is called **sickle cell disease.**

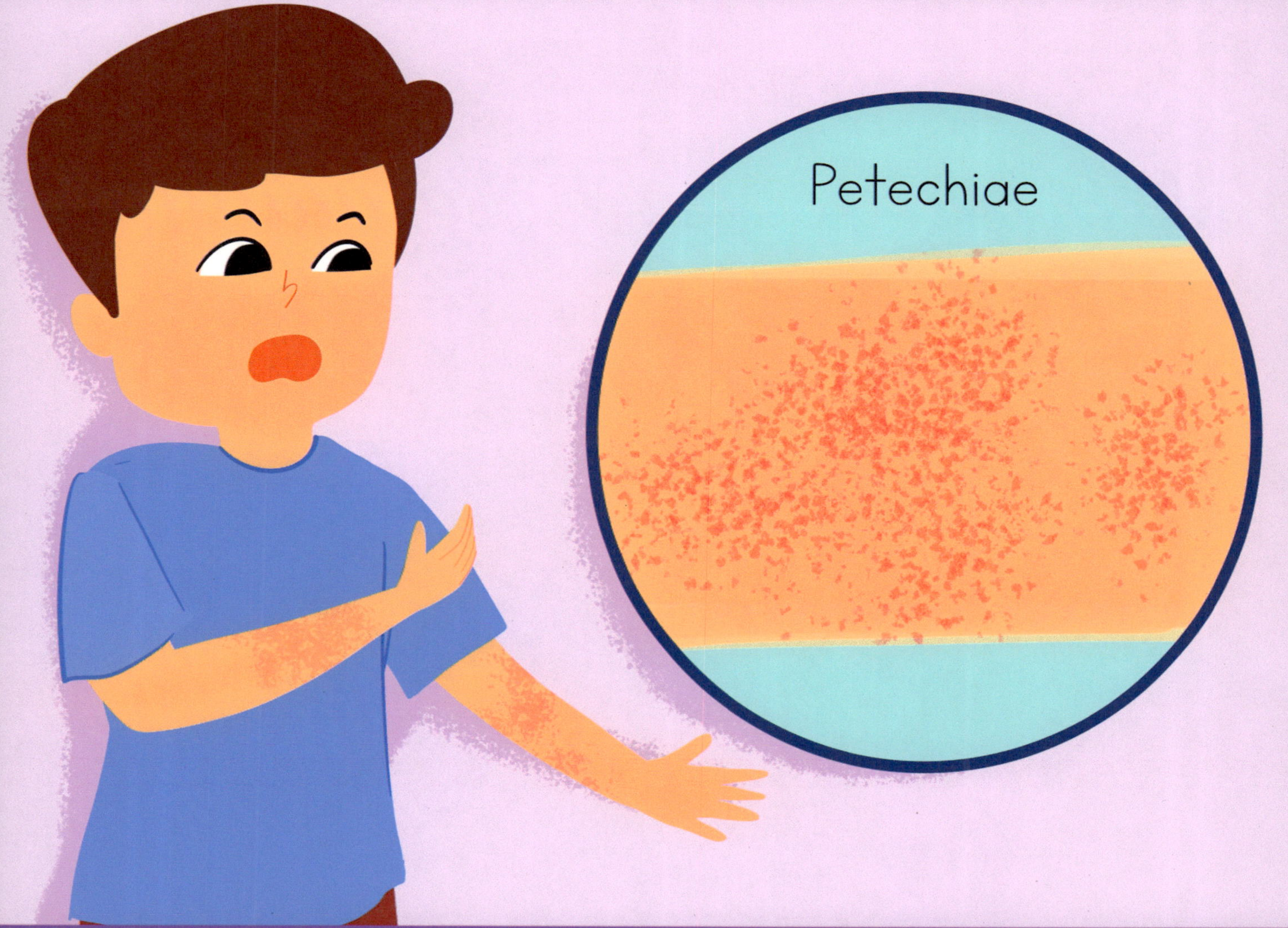

Having too few platelets is called **thrombocytopenia.** This can cause patients to bleed more easily and develop small red dots on their skin called **petechiae**.

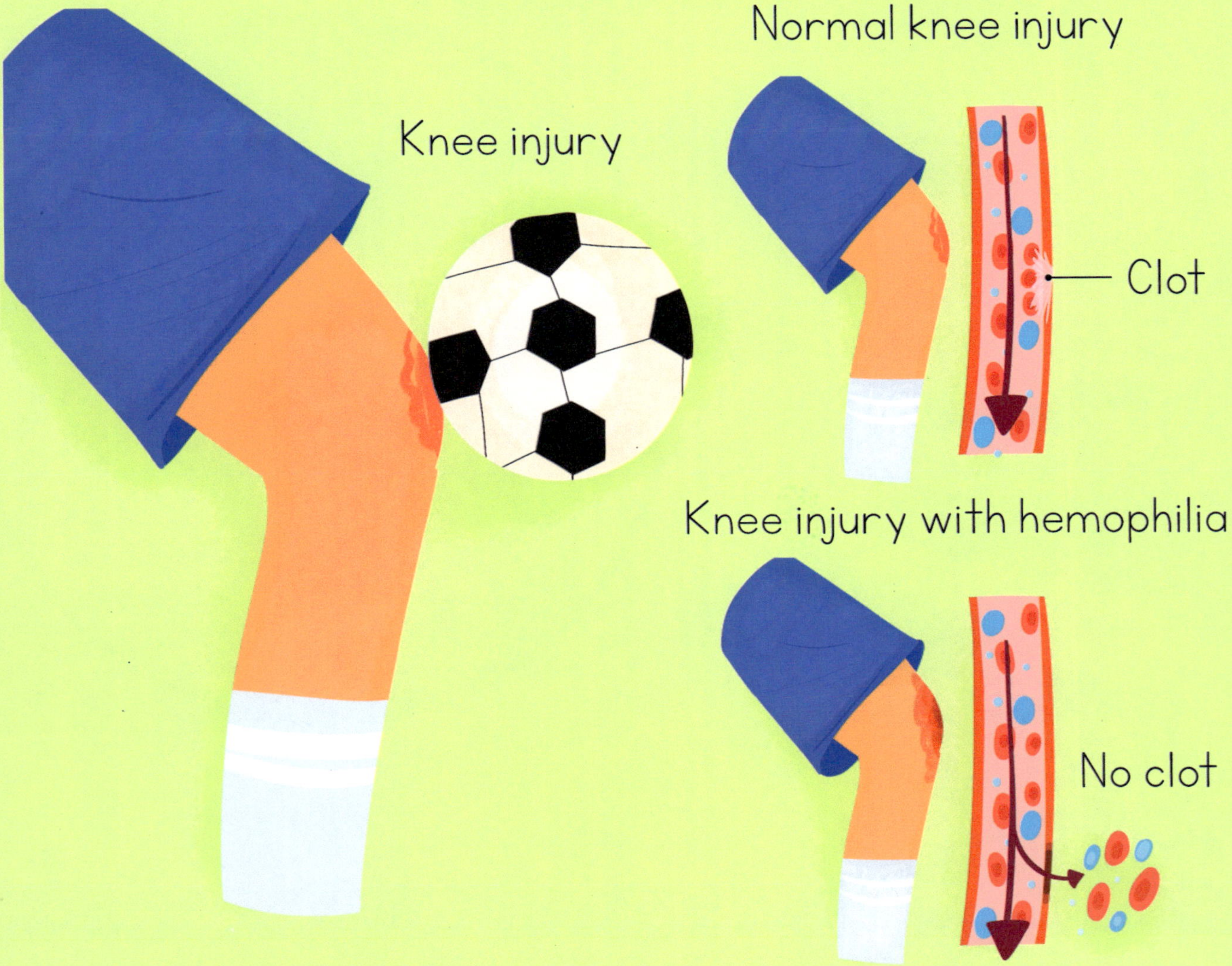

Some patients with a condition called **hemophilia** can also bleed more easily due to problems with clotting factors in their blood.

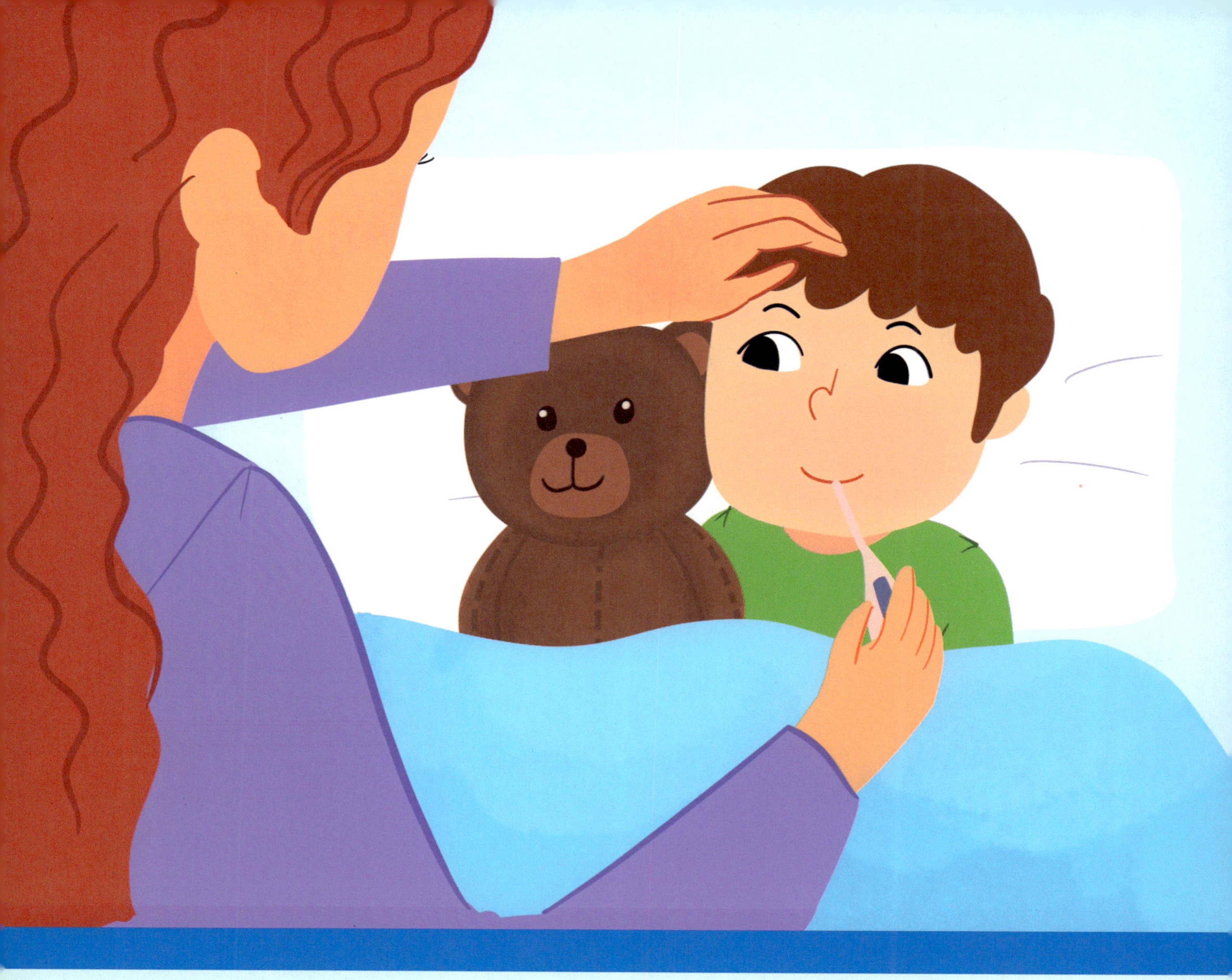

Having too few white blood cells is called **leukopenia**. This can cause patients to develop infections more easily.

Cancer development

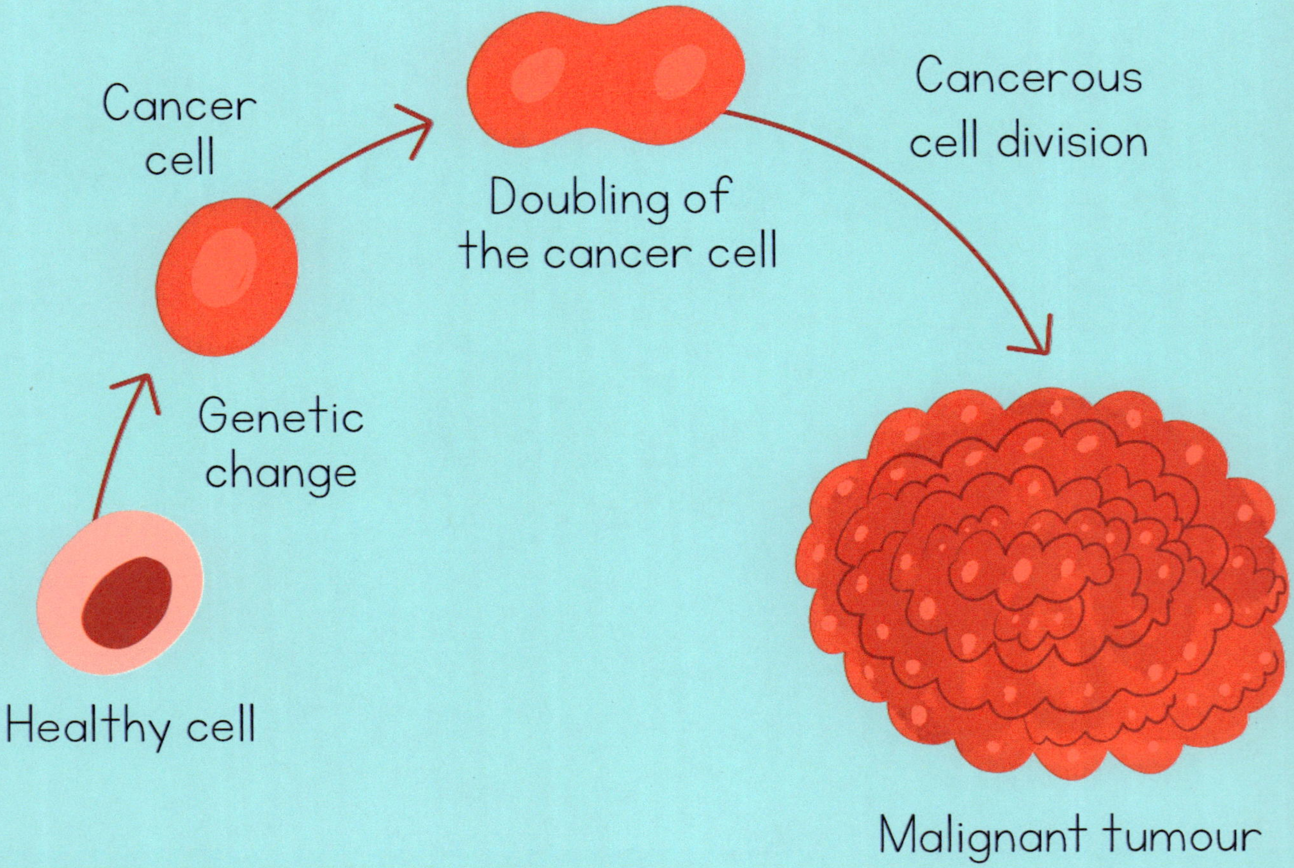

Other patients might have too *many* cells in their blood. This can occur if cells in their blood divide uncontrollably. This is called **cancer**.

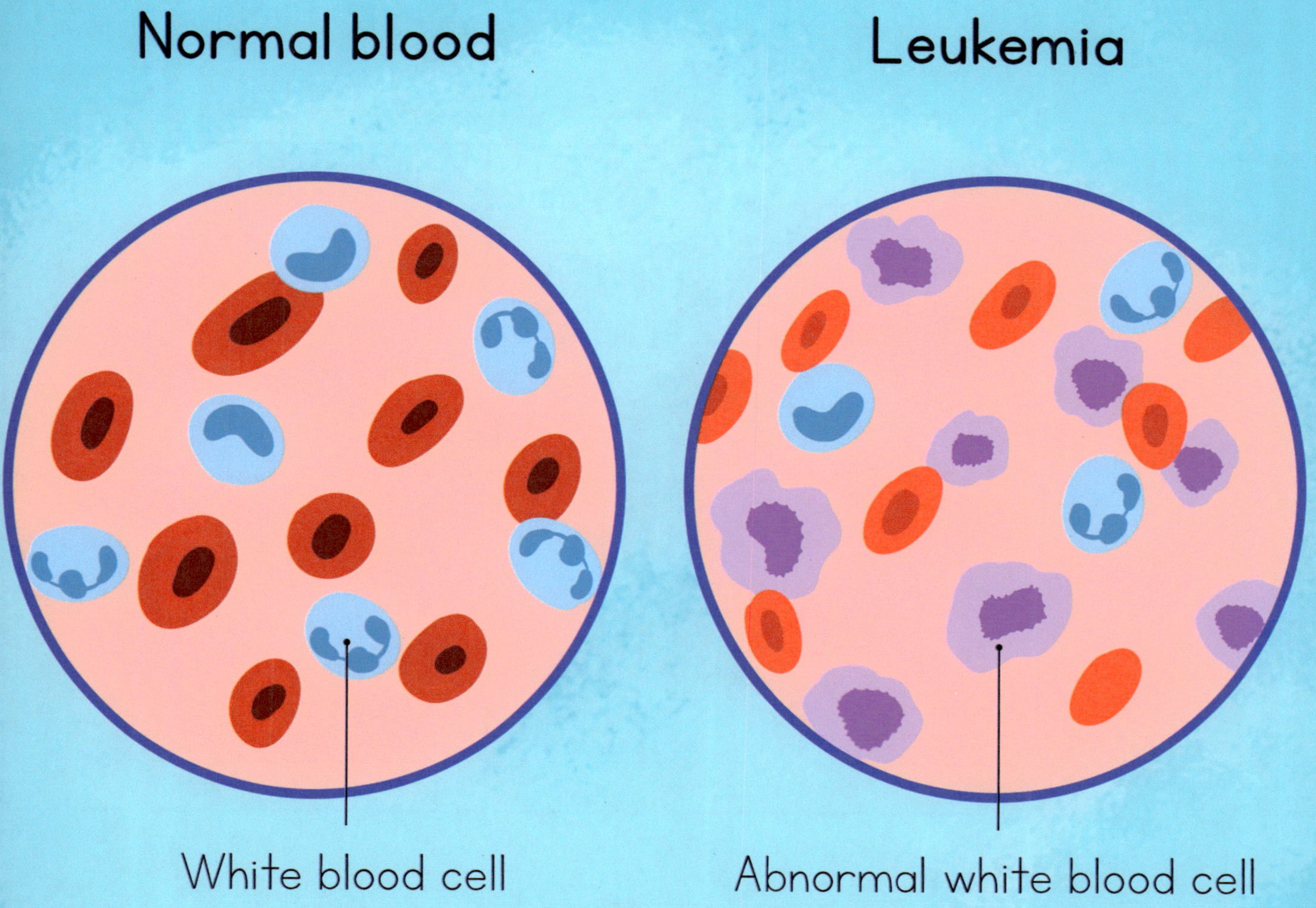

One type of cancer that can affect our blood is called **leukemia**. There are four main types of leukemia.

	Acute	Chronic
Myeloid	Acute myeloid leukemia (AML)	Chronic myeloid leukemia (CML)
Lymphocytic	Acute lymphocytic leukemia (ALL)	Chronic lymphocytic leukemia (CLL)

Acute myeloid leukemia and **acute lymphocytic leukemia** are fast-growing cancers. **Chronic myeloid leukemia** and **chronic lymphocytic leukemia** are slow-growing cancers.

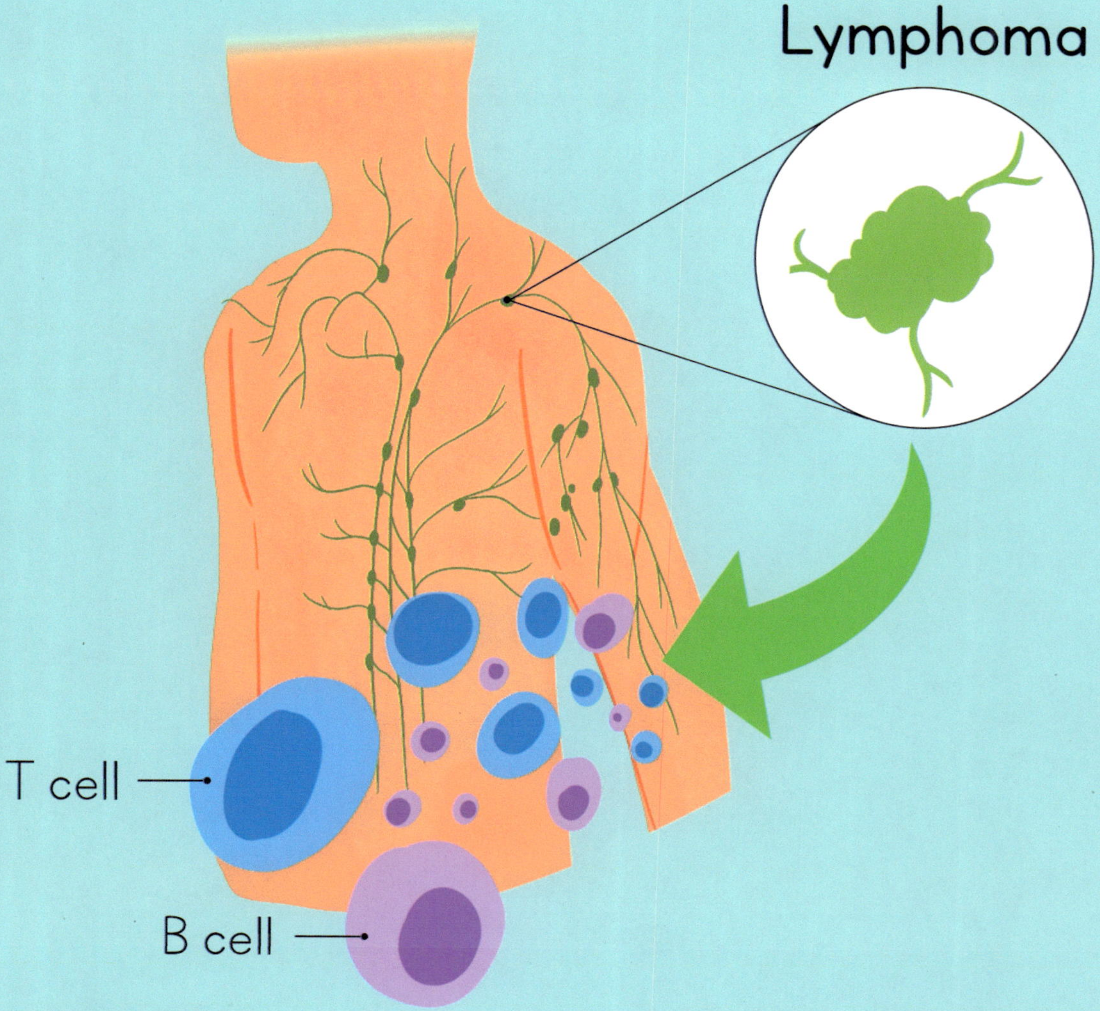

Another type of cancer that can affect our lymph nodes is called **lymphoma**. There are two main types of lymphoma.

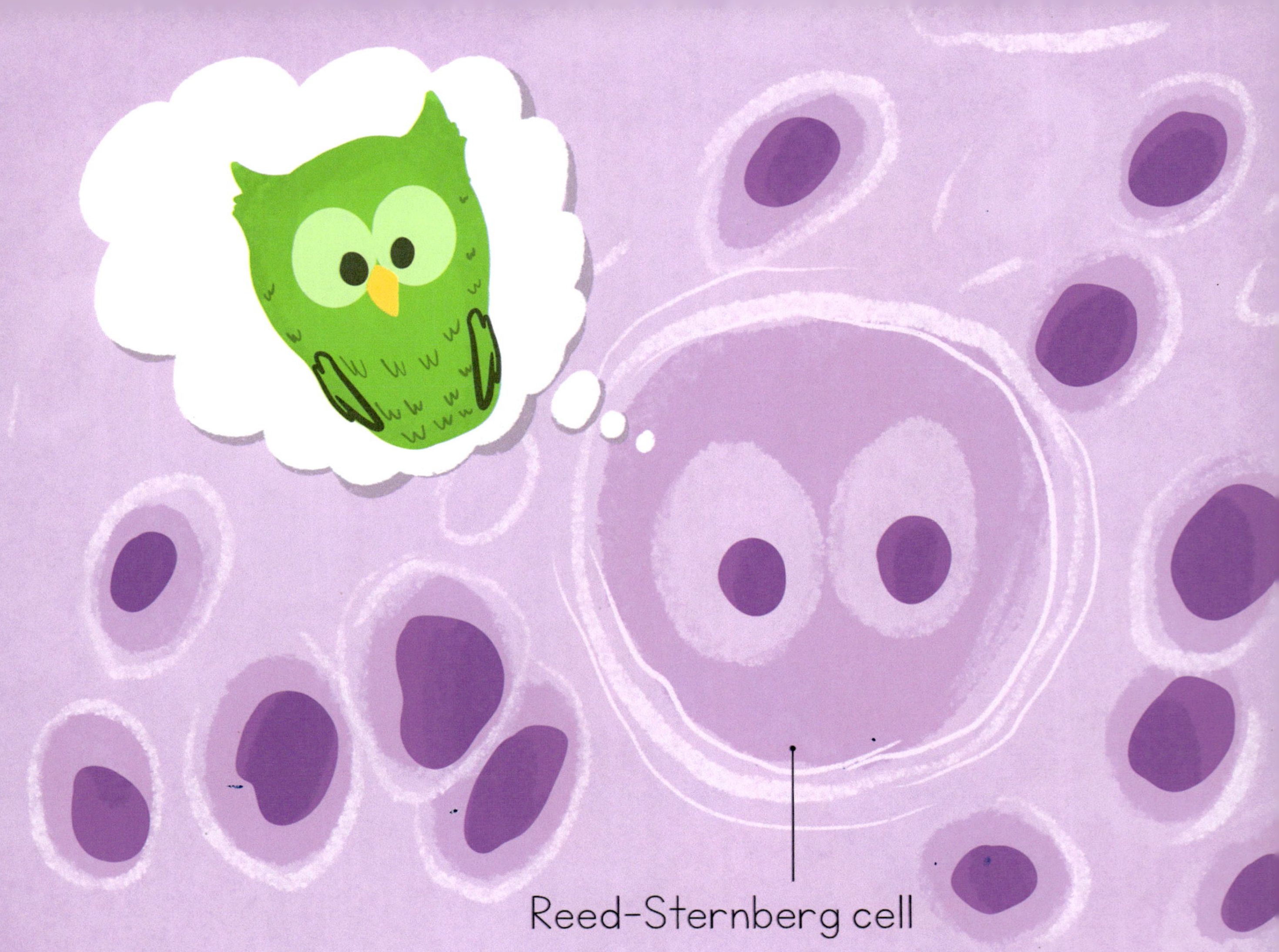

Hodgkin lymphoma has **Reed-Sternberg cells**, which look like owl eyes under a microscope, but **Non-Hodgkin lymphoma** does not.

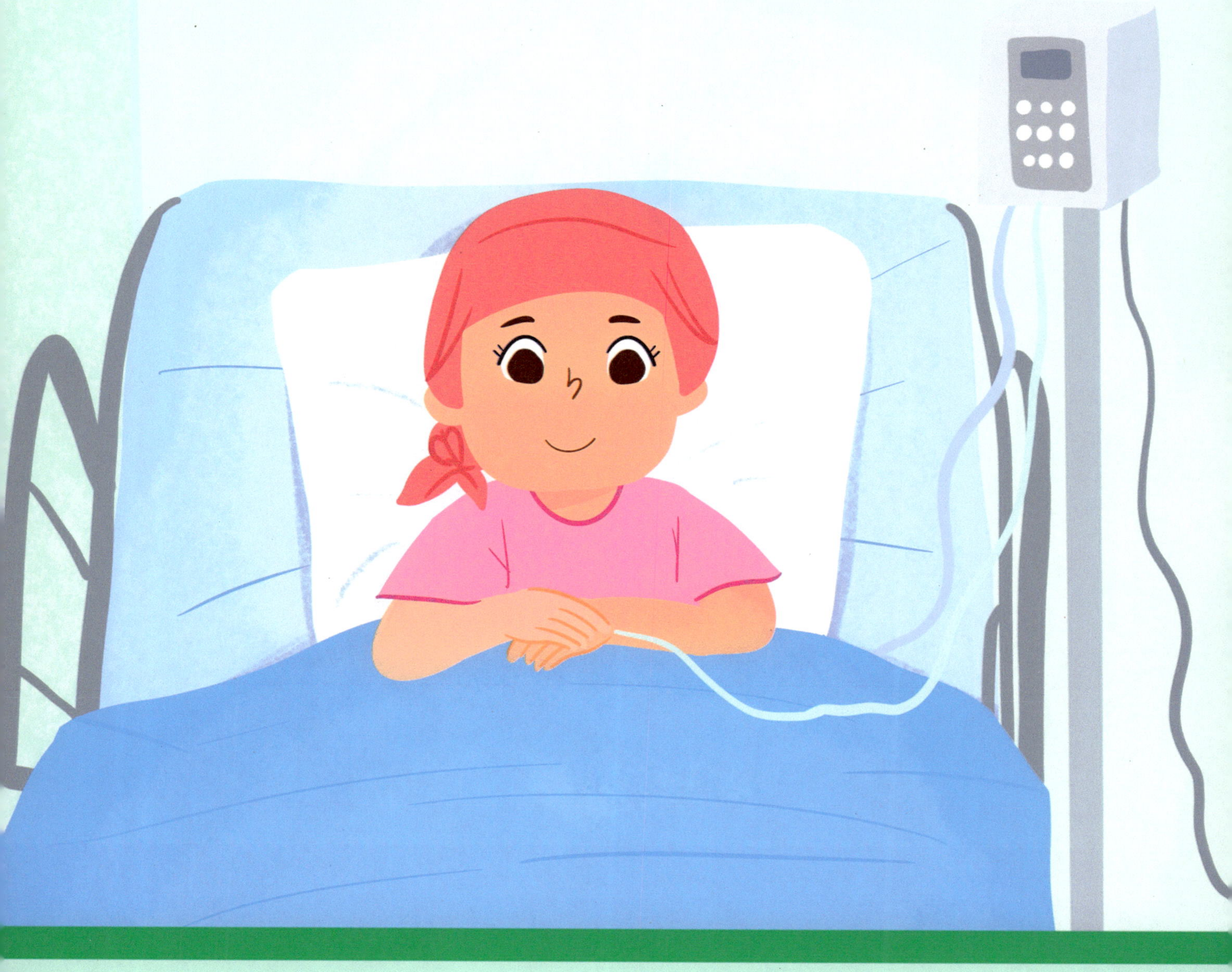

Fortunately, there are many treatments that can help patients with cancer get better!

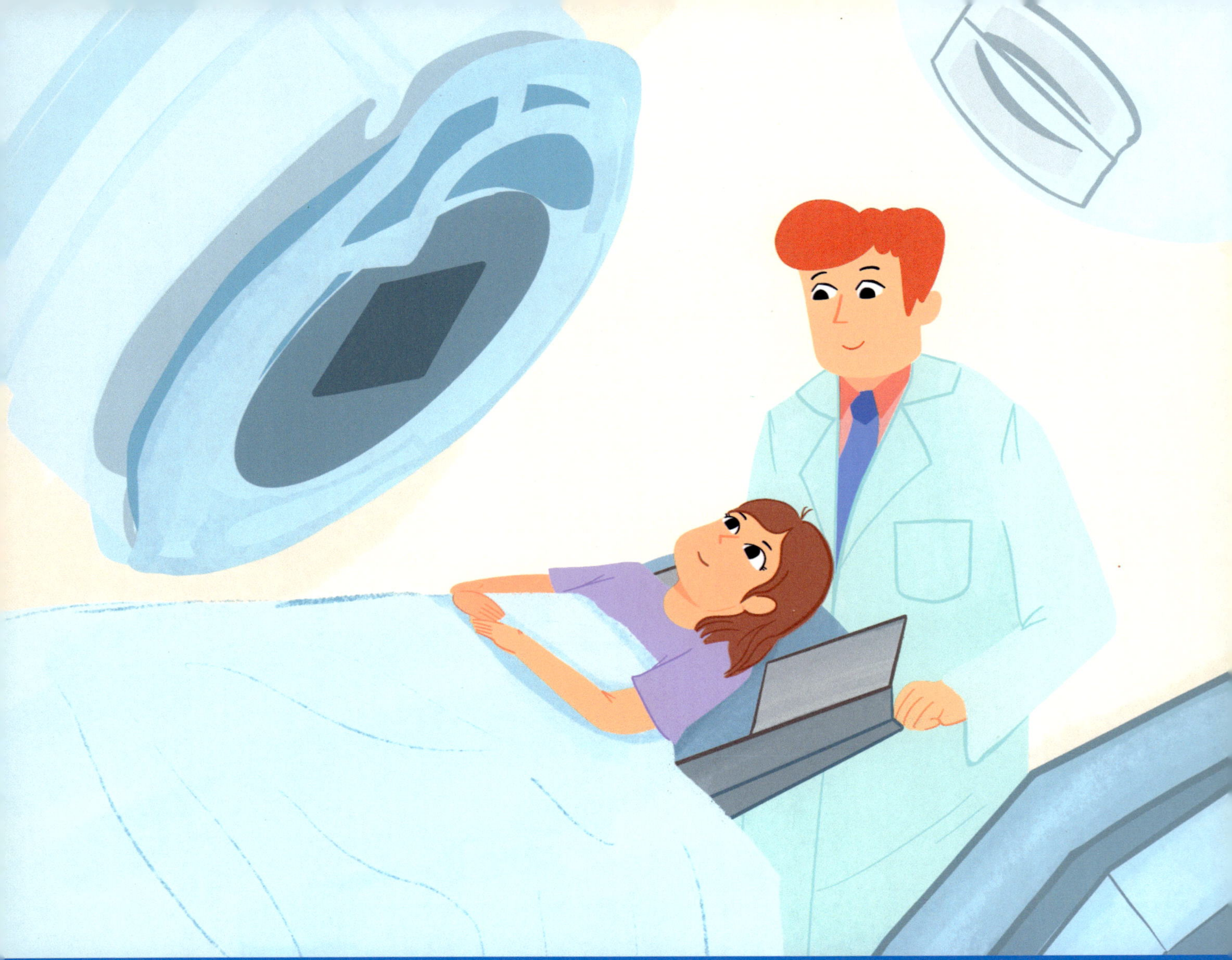

Radiation therapy uses a special type of light with a lot of energy to destroy cancer cells in specific areas of the body.

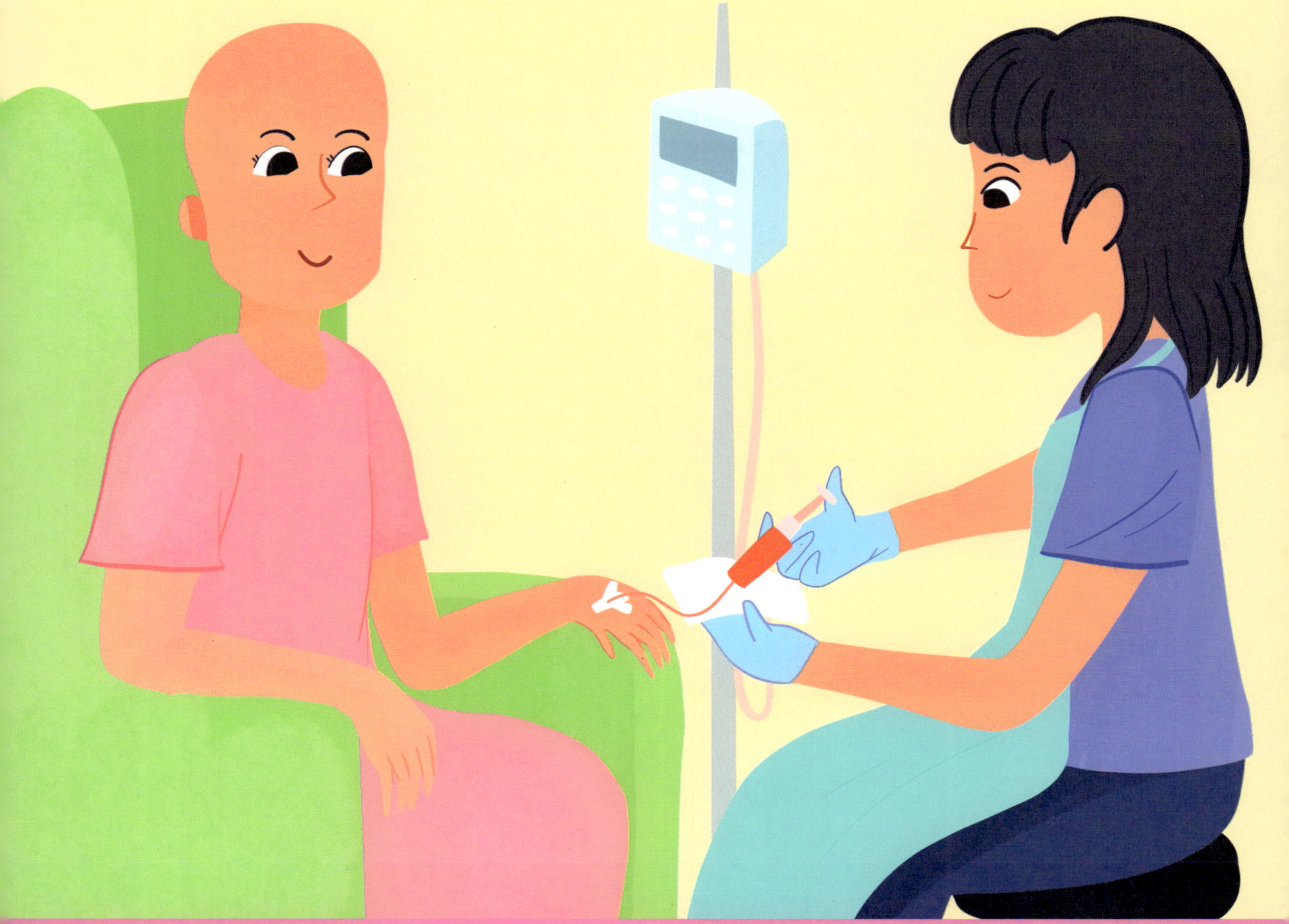

Chemotherapy uses special medications that stop or slow the growth of many different types of cells, including cancer, in the body.

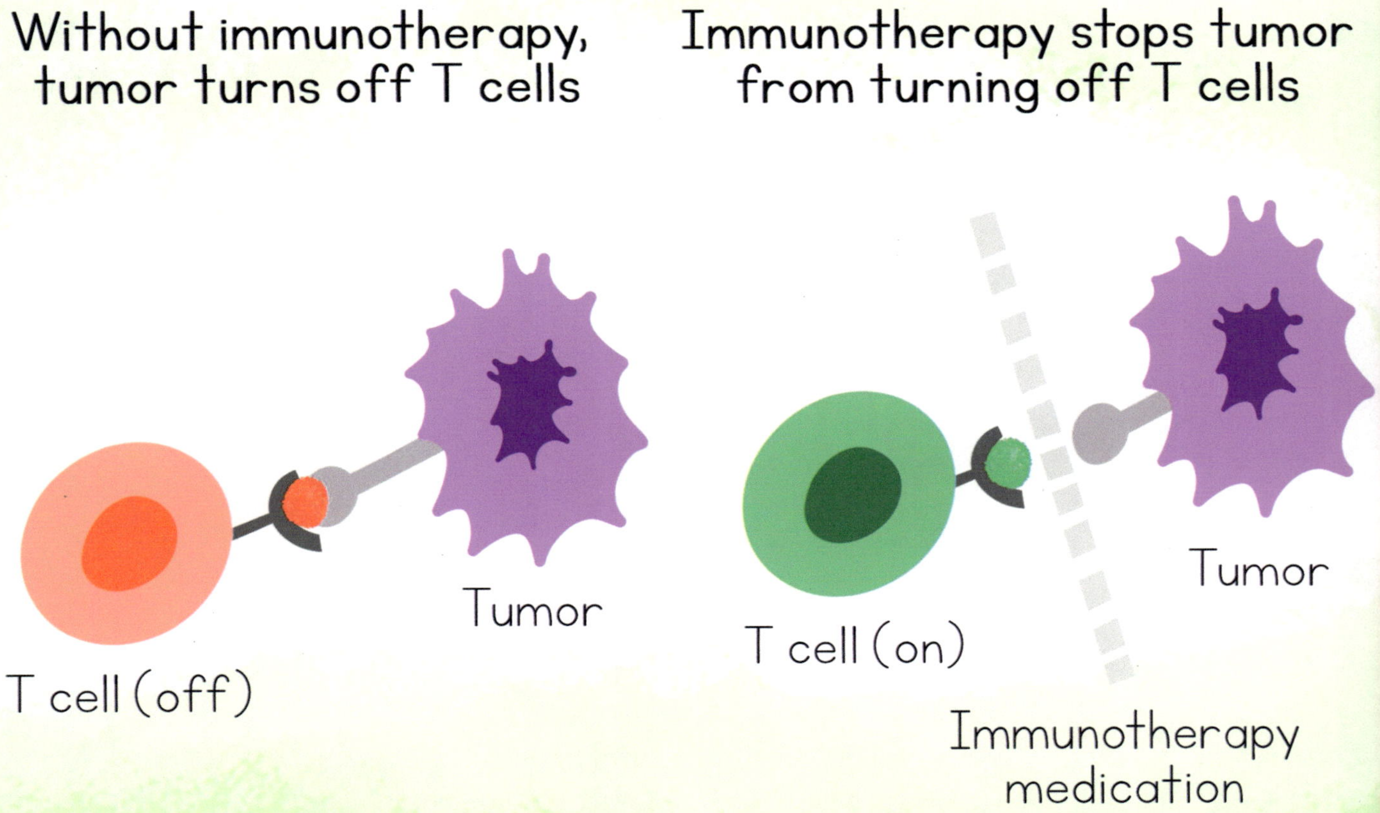

Immunotherapy uses special medications that help our immune system fight cancer cells. Some of these medications prevent cancer cells from blocking our immune system!

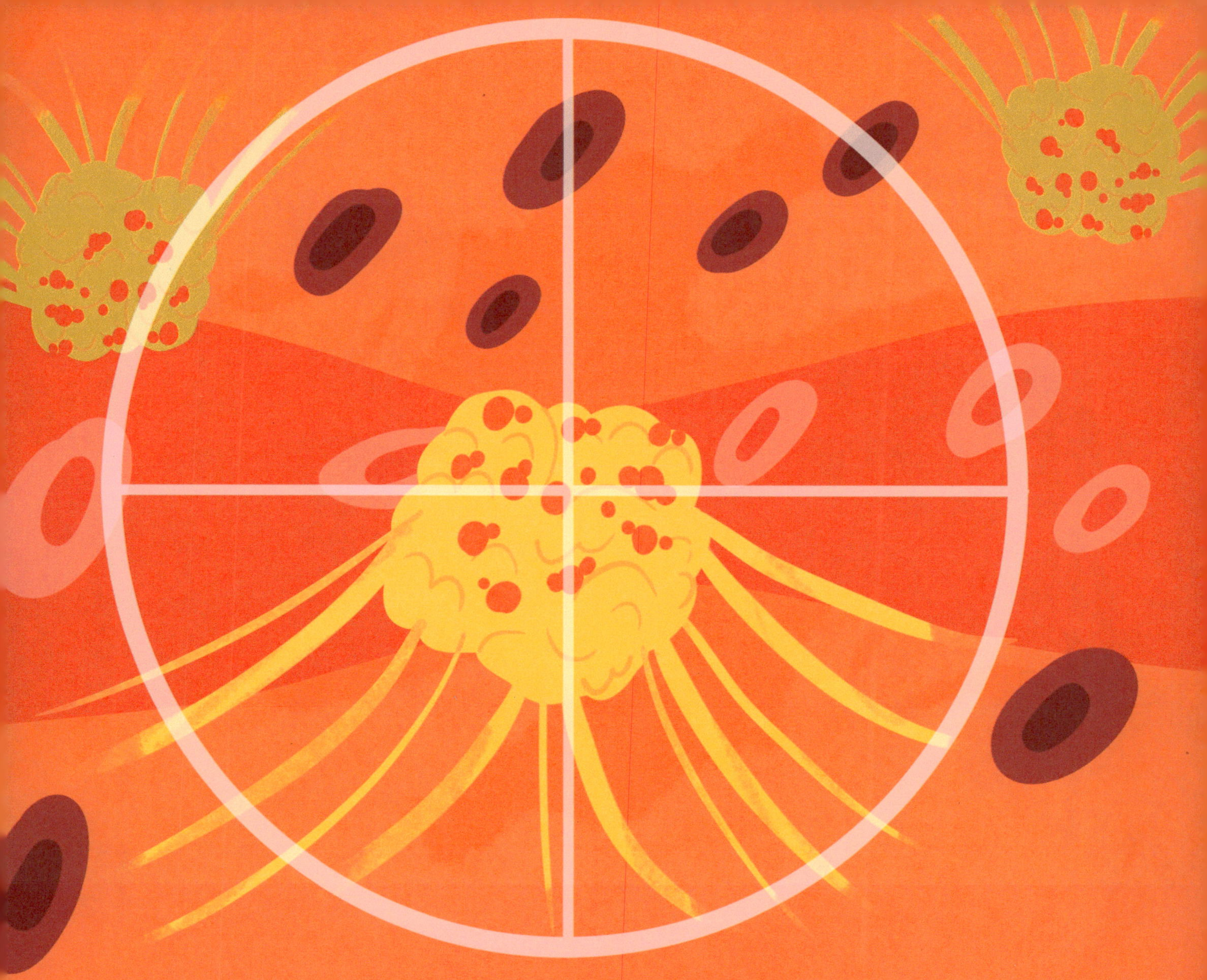

Targeted therapy uses medications that target and fight specific types of cancer cells.

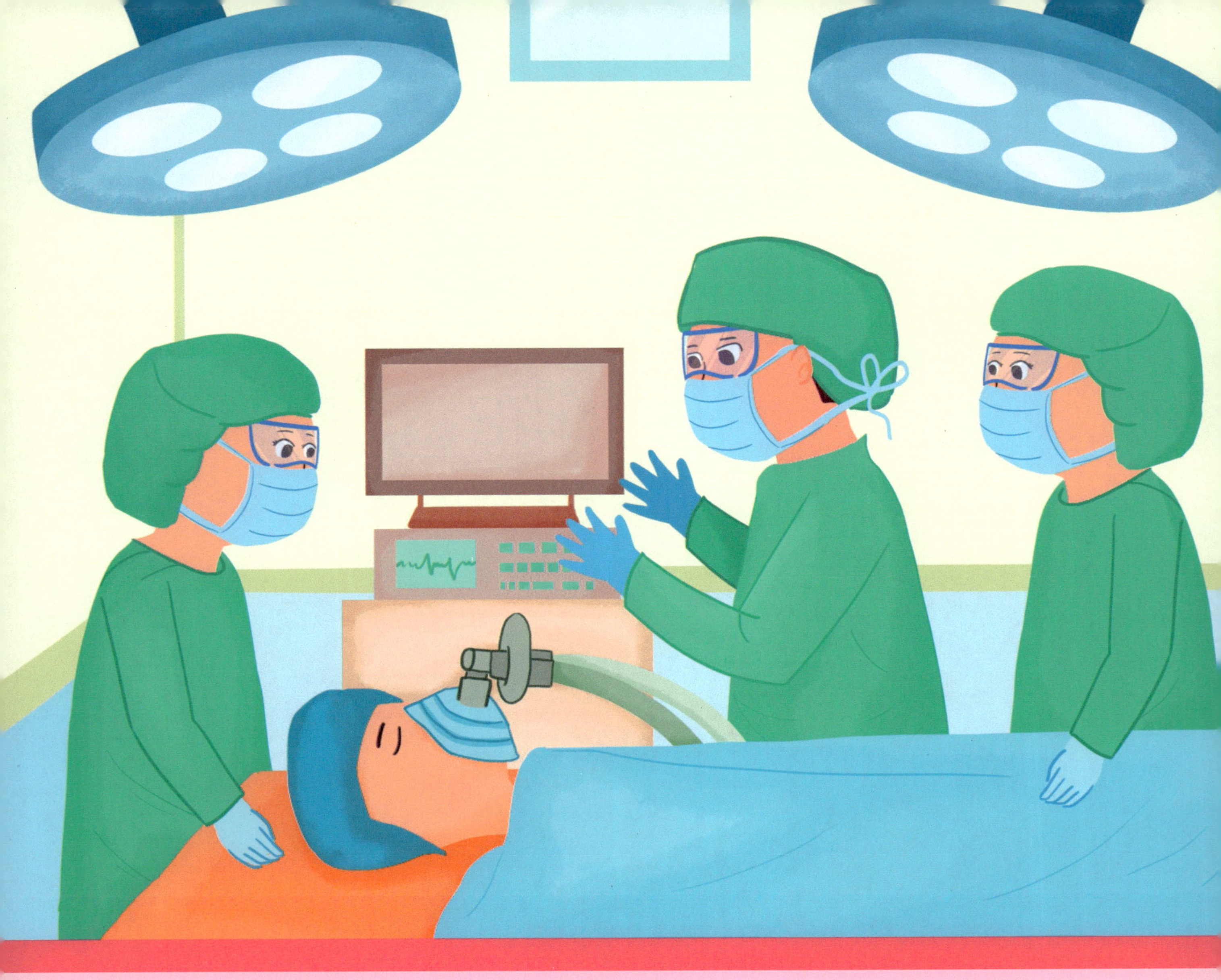

Patients with other types of cancer that affect their body's organs may undergo **surgery** to remove the cancer.

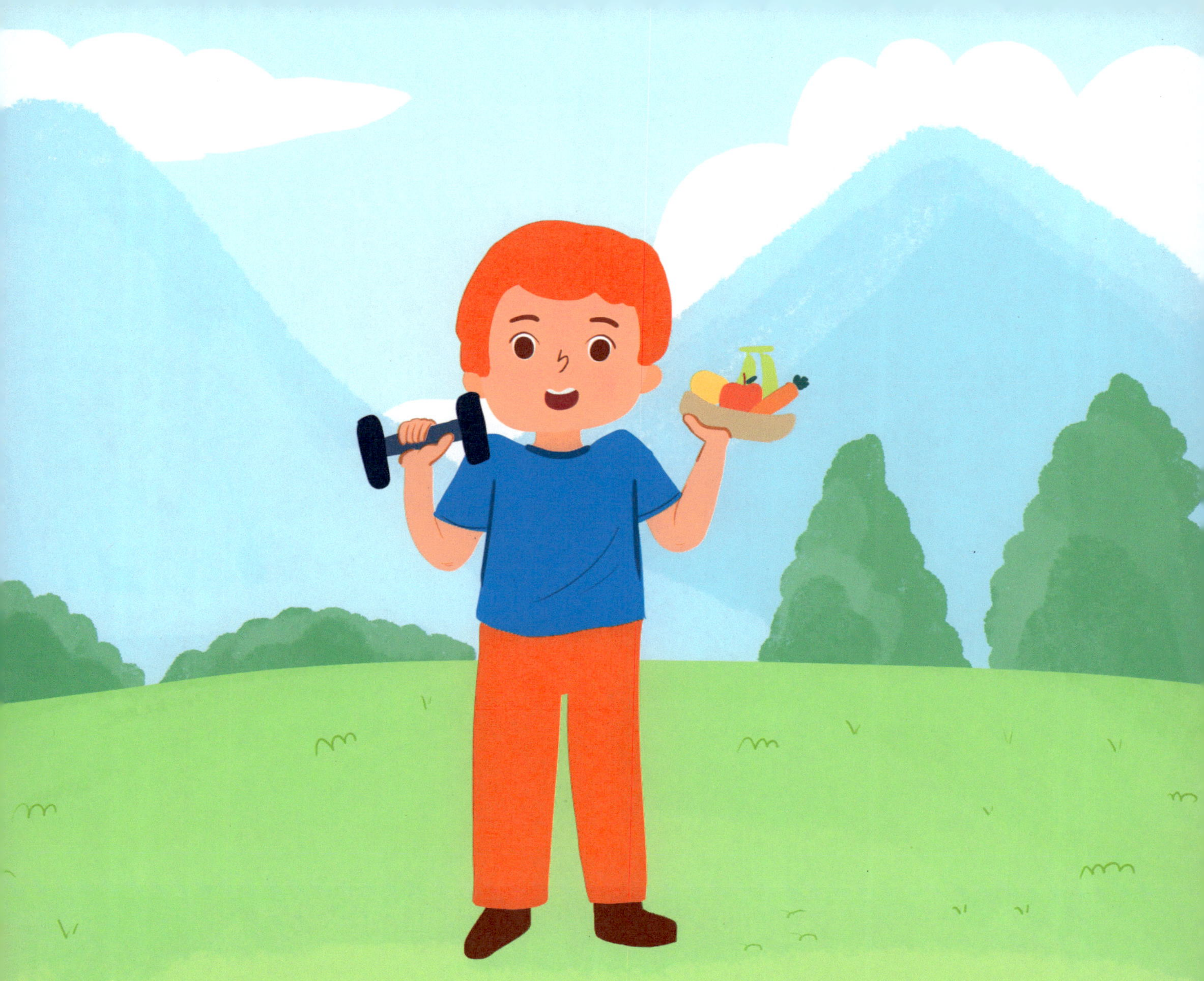

Exercising regularly and eating a balanced diet with plenty of fruits, vegetables, and whole grains can reduce our risk for cancer.

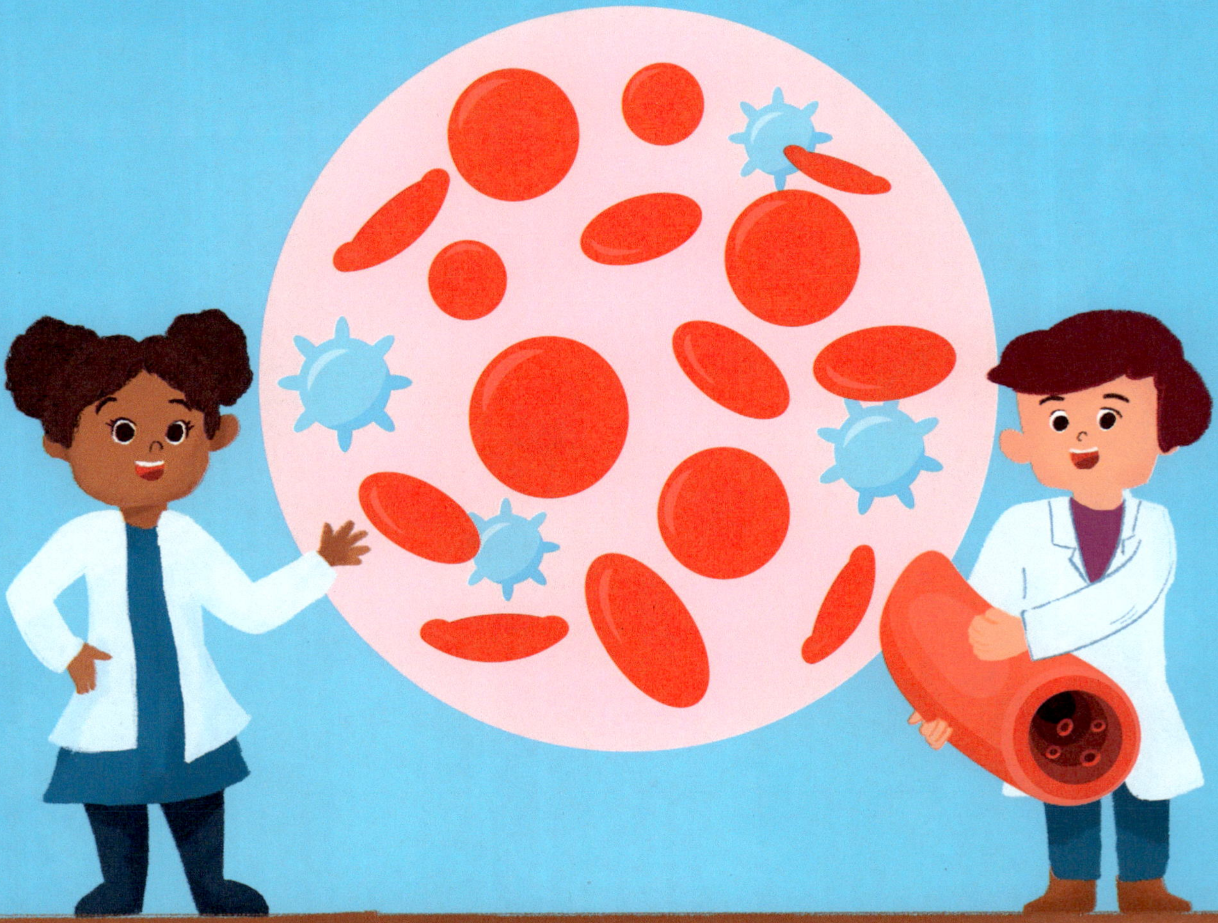

YOU'RE A FUTURE HEMATOLOGIST ONCOLOGIST!

Glossary

Anemia (uh-NEE-mee-uh): condition of having too few red blood cells; can be caused by **sickle cell disease** or deficiencies in **iron**, **folate**, or **vitamin B12**

Blood (bluhd): red fluid that travels through our blood vessels

Cancer (KAN-sr): condition in which cells in our body divide uncontrollably; **leukemia** is a cancer of the blood, and **lymphoma** is a cancer of lymph nodes

Chemotherapy (kee-moh-THEH-ruh-pee): special medications that stop or slow the growth of many types of cells, including cancer, in the body

Hematopoietic stem cell (hee-muh-toh-poi-ET-ik stem sel): immature cell that can develop into **red blood cells**, **platelets**, and **white blood cells**

Hemoglobin (HEE-moh-glow-bn): protein in red blood cells that binds to oxygen

Hemophilia (hee-moh-FEE-lee-uh): inherited bleeding disorder in which blood does not clot properly due to problems with clotting factors in the blood

Immunotherapy (i-myoo-noh-THEH-ruh-pee): special medications that help our immune system fight cancer cells

Leukopenia (loo-kow-PEE-nee-uh): condition of having too few white blood cells

Radiation therapy (ray-dee-AY-shn THEH-ruh-pee): treatment that uses a special type of light with a lot of energy to destroy cancer cells in specific areas

Targeted therapy (TAAR-guh-tuhd THEH-ruh-pee): special medications that target and fight specific types of cancer cells

Thrombocytopenia (thraam-buh-sai-tuh-PEE-nee-uh): condition of having too few platelets

Let's review what you learned!

1. Cells in our blood develop from what cells? Where are these cells located?
2. What are the three main types of cells in our blood?
3. What type of blood test can doctors use to look at these cells?
4. What is the job of red blood cells? Platelets? White blood cells?
5. What is the name of the protein in red blood cells that binds to oxygen?
6. What blood test can tell us the amounts of cells in our blood?
7. What is the name of the condition characterized by too few red blood cells? Too few platelets? Too few white blood cells?
8. Deficiencies in what three vitamins can lead to anemia?
9. What condition causes red blood cells to be crescent-shaped?
10. What condition can be caused by problems with clotting factors in the blood?
11. What is the name of a type of cancer that affects the blood?
12. What are the four main types of leukemia?
13. What is the name of a type of cancer that affects the lymph nodes?
14. What are the two main types of lymphoma?
15. What are four possible medical treatments for cancer?
16. What two things can we do to lead a healthy lifestyle and reduce our risk for cancer?

Medical School FOR KIDS™

Your Answers

1. ______________________________
2. ______________________________
3. ______________________________
4. ______________________________
5. ______________________________
6. ______________________________
7. ______________________________
8. ______________________________
9. ______________________________
10. ______________________________
11. ______________________________
12. ______________________________
13. ______________________________
14. ______________________________
15. ______________________________
16. ______________________________

Medical School FOR KIDS™

Answer Key

1. Hematopoietic stem cells; bone marrow
2. Red blood cells, platelets, and white blood cells
3. Blood smear
4. To transport oxygen from our lungs to the rest of our body; to prevent and stop bleeding; to fight infections and other diseases
5. Hemoglobin
6. Complete blood count (CBC)
7. Anemia; thrombocytopenia; leukopenia
8. Iron, folate, vitamin B12
9. Sickle cell disease
10. Hemophilia
11. Leukemia
12. Acute myeloid leukemia, acute lymphocytic leukemia, chronic myeloid leukemia, and chronic lymphocytic leukemia
13. Lymphoma
14. Hodgkin lymphoma and non-Hodgkin lymphoma
15. Radiation therapy, chemotherapy, immunotherapy, and targeted therapy
16. Exercise regularly and eat a balanced diet with plenty of healthy foods

Medical School FOR KIDS™

About the Authors

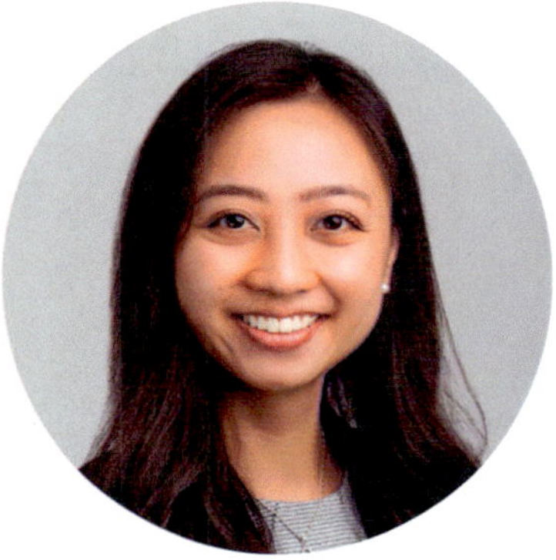

Betty Nguyen, MD

Betty is a physician specializing in dermatology at the University of Miami. She was born in Southern California but spent much of her childhood in Georgia, where she grew up on a chicken farm. Betty studied Biology at UCLA, where she was a Gates Millennium Scholar, and earned her MD from UC Riverside on a full-tuition scholarship. Outside of work, Betty is a certified yoga instructor and licensed scuba diver. She also enjoys journalistic writing and cycling.

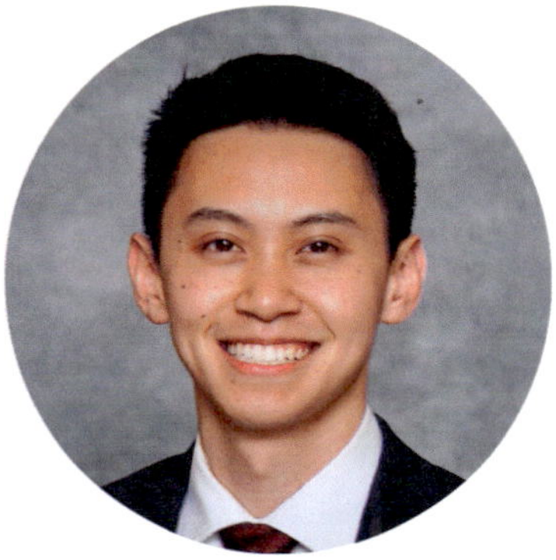

Brandon Pham, MD

Brandon is a physician specializing in ophthalmology at the Bascom Palmer Eye Institute in Miami. He was born and raised in Southern California. Brandon studied Microbiology, Immunology, and Molecular Genetics at UCLA, where he was a Barry Goldwater Scholar, and earned his MD from Stanford. He is passionate about medical education for students of all ages. In his free time, Brandon enjoys traveling, playing tennis, and performing card magic tricks.

Check out the rest of the books in our series!

Website: mdforkids.org

Instagram: @md.for.kids

Medical School FOR KIDS™

Made in the USA
Monee, IL
05 November 2026

67381728R00024